The Roadmap

Melting the Fear of Breast Cancer

Conventional & Naturopathic Choices

By Joe & Laura Patrina

Copyright © 2020 by J.A. Patrina.
Issued By Managing Breast Cancer LLC.

All rights reserved. No part of this book may be reproduced in any form or by any electronic or mechanical means, including information storage and retrieval systems, without permission in writing from the publisher, except by reviewers, who may quote brief passages in a review.

ISBN: 978-1-7330672-6-3   [Paperback Edition]

Printed and bound in The United States of America.

Published by LittleHouse Enterprises Inc.

THE ROADMAP
Laura's Note

This book – "The Roadmap – Melting the Fear of Breast Cancer" – outlines ideas coming out of both conventional and naturopathic medicine. It prepares you for discussions with the diversity of clinical experts you will interact with.

As described on the ManagingBreastCancer.com web site, based upon our personal journey with breast cancer starting in 2014 onwards, my husband Joe and I realized that no web site was available to organize the hundreds of *Conventional Medicine* and *Naturopathic* topics arising out of both worlds.

As a result, when I received my diagnosis, we suddenly found ourselves adrift in the unknown, with no way to counter our fear. We craved information, but found it scattered across the internet, plus the treatment doctors we met only spoke from within their individual silos of expertise.

For some time, we lived in a state of deep dread.

But as our research slowly uncovered countermeasures to the disease, we began to shed these layers of dread. Days of worry were replaced with a determination to add to our budding list of self-healing measures.

We soon understood how cancer starts, how long it takes to become visible, the nutrients it craves, the tricks it plays with inflammation and angiogenesis enzymes, its acidic/no-oxygen comfort zone, and the things that dismantle its comfort zone. We also came to understand the role of aging, the accumulation of toxins after many decades, the age-related changes that weaken the bodies resolve, and the supplements that at least partially restore this resolve.

We then realized that most of these measures ought apply to prevention starting in one's 30's, and that even after receiving conventional treatment, prevention again is called for to hold the fort. The peak age for breast cancer is in one's mid-sixties, but many cases fall on either side of that curve, and many instances of new outbreaks can plague women across many decades.

So, as is said "stay woke", but in this case the "stay woke" topics focus upon health-enhancements and tactical-countermeasures. Just come armed with this know-how to provide emotional ballast for your little ship.

Getting cancer is a wake-up call demonstrating that you can no longer take things for granted. Action is needed. Even if you outsource some of this action to conventional doctors, it does not relieve you from getting educated and for you to do whatever you can to optimize your future.

That is where ManagingBreastCancer.com – "The Resource Center" comes in. There, you can quickly become educated, and can even drill down deeply by enrolling in the site's Master Class video series. And with both feet on the ground, you can formulate a unified plan that taps into both the Conventional Medicine and Naturopathic worlds.

Plus, many of the women we have spoken with say that they would appreciate access to support people well versed in the subject matter. This support service is described on the *ManagingBreastCancer.com* web site.

READ THIS FIRST

Disclaimer

ROADMAP is not a formula to cure cancer. It is an assembly of ideas coming out of the naturopathic community describing how to bolster one's health, which may be of value when confronting cancer. No claim is cited as proven. Assertions are solely internal views on the possible explanations of why some actions may work. We share these personal insights with you merely as background and not as a prescription. Use your own best counsel and judgement - including discussions with cancer medical doctor specialists - in any course of action taken regarding your health.

THE BOOKS & THE MASTER CLASS VIDEOS

As described, to quickly get women up to speed on prevention and treatment topics, the authors envisioned a breast cancer resource center that brought together information coming out of both Conventional Medicine and Naturopathic fields. After seven years of research the Breast Cancer Resource Center was launched in 2021, offering:

Guides, White Papers, Books, Master Class Videos, Blog TV Segments, and One-on-one Coaching.

The optic? "Replace fear with perspective, but don't go it alone."

By 2021, our multi-year educational run resulted in four published resources.

THE ROADMAP – Melting the Fear of Breast Cancer

This synopsis of our findings is a guide book to get you started. Its goal, *to replace fear with perspective*. We want you to approach the subject in a levelheaded manner.

THE MASTERCLASS – A Video Education Program

This 35 video course program teaches the naturopath measures that one can incorporate into a personal self-healing plan. The program describes a take action blueprint on over 30 health-boosting measures that may prevent and reverse cancer, and that can complement conventional treatment.

DEFEATING BREAST CANCER – No Surgery, Chemotherapy or Radiation

This detailed 320-page *journal* follows Laura's journey to shrink her tumors solely using naturopathic means. Learn how the authors uncovered treatment options and how they weathered the emotional storm.

THE LIBRARY – Free Essays found on the ManagingBreastCancer.com web site

This ongoing set of short essays covers many important topics. One can sign up to receive new releases as they are published. Examples include:

- What Happens Once Diagnosed
- How Cancer Evolves
- Tumor Development Timeframes
- A Chemotherapy Brief
- A Radiation Brief
- Contraceptives & Breast Cancer
- Naturopathic FAQs
- A Prevention Outline

All four publications are of great value for women suddenly confronted by the disease and the complex medical world that treats it.

Once you have digested the written material and watched the Master Class videos, the support service can be structured to help you move forward.

THE
ManagingBreastCancer.com
WEB SITE

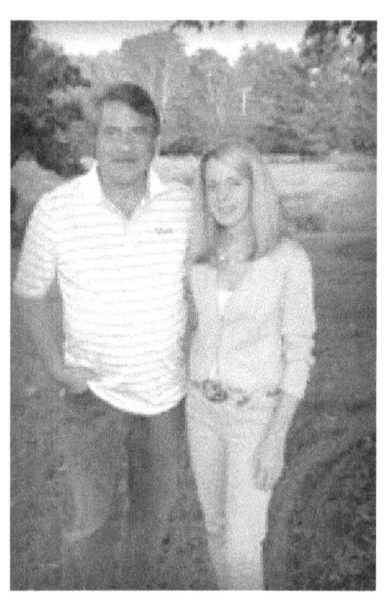

You can find the publications, videos and other short, free essays on the *ManagingBreastCancer.com*. web site.

For example, one important essay describes the types of Breast Cancer, another describes the time frames and stages of tumor development, and another prevention steps – starting in one's 30s.

Once you become acclimated to this new world of information, we advise that you move up to the *Master Class Program* video series. It is designed to keep you grounded as you implement some or all of the naturopathic measures.

We wish you the best and hope you can replace fear with perspective.

Joe & Laura

ROADMAP FAQS
To Get You Started

What's the single big idea? – For women to make the right choices in how to fight breast cancer, they need to know the ins and outs of *both* traditional medicine and naturopathic solutions.

What are the traditional medicine options? – *Lumpectomies*, where part of the breast is removed, *mastectomies* where the whole breast is removed, *radiation* where the breast and armpit lymph nodes are ionized to disrupt other occurrences of the cancer, and *chemotherapy*, a poison sickening all cells, configured to hurt cancer cells the worst. Traditional options boil down to actions that cut, burn and poison to kill cancer as soon as possible.

What are the naturopathic solutions? Any measure that spurs the body to heal itself, things like diet, nutritional supplements, immune system boosters, circulatory and digestive aids, and lifestyle changes that offset decades of aging.

What is meant by holistic and homeopathic? "Holistic" simply means treating the whole body using *naturopathic* actions to cure even just one component of the body. "Homeopathic" is a specific naturopathic technique which uses the very poison making you sick (say mercury), to draw out buried poison trapped inside your cells. Advocates call it "Like cures like". Homeo = like, Pathic = Disease.

What are the supporting ideas? – Breast cancer develops over a period of 6 to 10 years. There are naturopathic steps one can take to thwart cancer at each phase of its development, starting with prevention actions taken in one's 30s, extending to arresting advanced conditions which usually manifest themselves any time after age 45 (the medium age is in one 60's).

What are today's societal norms? – Habitually, terrified women are left without choice and rushed into surgery, and then given radiation and/or chemo and reconstructive surgery. Women need to be educated about ALL the options, both prevention oriented and healing oriented. Imagine tackling a cancer diagnosis FEAR FREE!

What surprises people? – That one can fight the cancer on one's own terms, exploring naturopathic options, learning how to monitor the results. Dread can be replaced with knowledge and management.

Who is affected? – Every single day matters with breast cancer. One-in-seven women will be diagnosed at some point in their life, with 280,000 new cases a year surfacing in the U.S. alone. But because it takes 6 to 10 years for tumors to become visible, much can be done to stem their advance.

What are the trends? – A growing cultural trend seeks alternatives. As people shun the devastation of surgery, chemotherapy and radiation, explanations are sought for naturopathic approaches. Thankfully - more-and-more - traditional doctors and scientists are joining to provide these answers.

What are the top mistakes made in fighting breast cancer? – Instead of visualizing a break-down in one's overall cellular health, many assume cancer a foreign aberration. And some believe naturopathic options remain "pop medicine", unable to be proven. As a result, people freeze, doing nothing to stem root causes at the cellular level.

What are some faulty beliefs? – 5-year survival statistics ignore re-occurrences, and leave the impression that percentages apply across one's total remaining years. Handing your fate over to medical intervention for 5-year promises does not get you off the hook.

What are the most dangerous myths? – That you have no time. That cancer needs to be removed immediately otherwise life itself is risked. That modern chemotherapy and radiation treatments are markedly better than before, causing less damage. That the death-by-cancer statistic as a percentage of the population has improved; it has remained constant since World War II.

What contrarian idea matters most? That in navigating your health with proper knowhow, one can take matters into one's own hands. *And more, that having common sense does not require a medical degree.* Knowledge - when to work on your own and when to enlist medical specialists - represents true choice. But to navigate a cancer diagnosis, one needs to come armed with knowhow.

Why was *ManagingBreastCancer.com* – *The Resource Center* assembled? Most importantly to navigate the FEAR of a diagnosis. There are many moving parts towards confronting breast cancer. The books, the white papers and The Master Class video course program organize a wide foundation of information, giving women intellectual and emotional ballast.

Contents

FAQs ix
Introduction xiv
Phase 1: Healthy Cells – In One's Youth 1
Phase 2: Assaulted Cells 5
Phase 3: Infected 11
Phase 4: Converted 17
Phase 5: Tumor Formed 22
Phase 6: Aggression 38
Phase 7 : Dominance 45
Phase 8: Metastasis 48

Supplement Appendix 51
Epilogue 62

INTRODUCTION

Age and deficits in health underpin cancer. And even if current tumors are removed or killed, one wants to do something to fix factors that might lead to new outbreaks. This life-long view is where naturopathic actions enter the conversation.

The naturopathic framework for rehabilitating your health includes:

1. *Diet* - Remove the glucose dietary supply and the inflammation stimulants that keep tumor growth aggressive.

2. *Infiltration* – Surround and infiltrate the tumor with things that confuse its division rates.

3. *Empowerment* - Strengthen the immune system so that this powerhouse army stymies colony formations.

Overall, we want to take tumors out of their comfort zone by changing one's health environment.

Organizationally, to present the detail in context, THE ROADMAP links specific naturopathic countermeasures to each respective cancer expansion phase – starting with how to bolster healthy cells, how to impede developing tumors, and how to slow metastasis.

For easy reference, specific product supplements mentioned along the way are listed in the appendix.

For some people, naturopathic countermeasures alone might lead to tumor reversal, as they did with Laura, the author (described in the Defeating Breast Cancer book). But many will elect to pursue a hybrid, incorporating naturopathic rehabilitation in conjunction with chemo, surgery and radiation to optimize one's chance of beating the disease now and over time.

THE ROADMAP will look at the eight (8) stages of cancer proliferation, and identify the countermeasures pertaining to each phase. As is obvious, most of the countermeasures can be followed for prevention purposes as well.

Regarding prevention, an outline on what to do in one's 30', 40's and beyond can be found in the *ManagingBreastCancer.com* on-line library.

The Eight Cancer Expansion Phases At the Cellular Level

1. Healthy	2. Assaulted
Oxygen, Nutrients, Hormone Support, Immune Support	Low Oxygen, Free Radicals, Nutrient Deficient, Low Immune Support
3. Infected	4. Converted
Viruses!	DNA Copy, Switched To Cancer Options, Divide Only Signals

Breast Cancer — The Roadmap

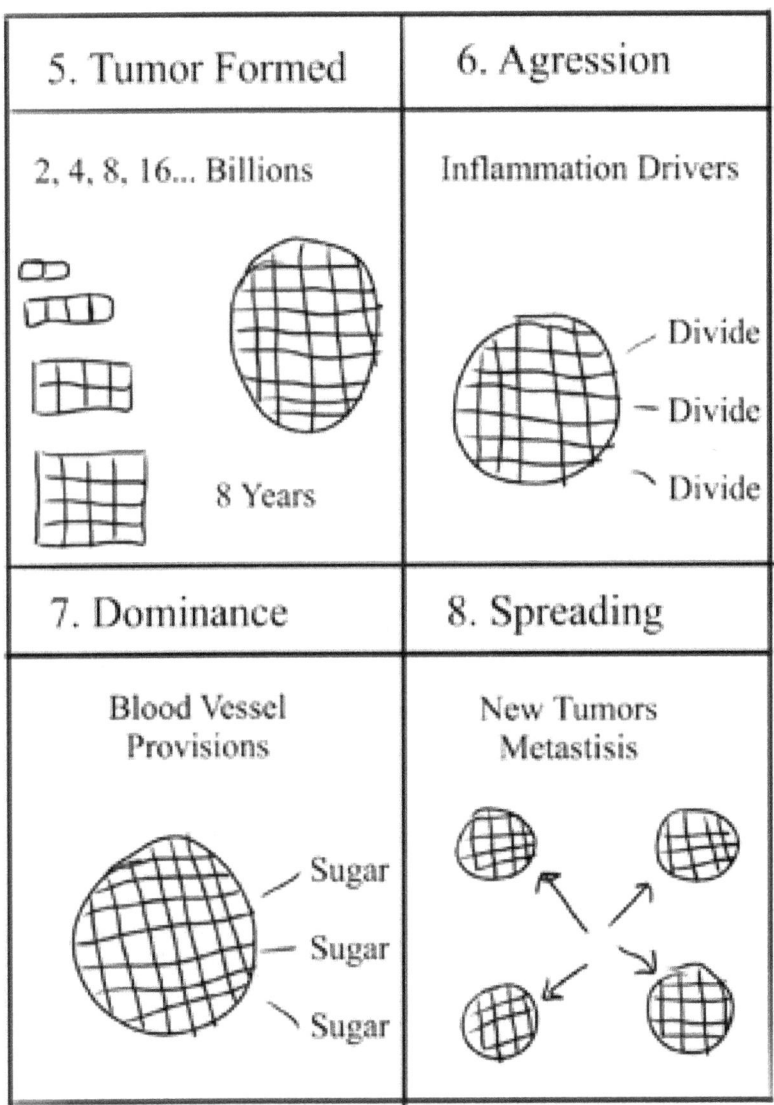

Phase 1
Healthy Cells – In One's Youth

For most people, during youth, their trillions of bodily cells remain healthy, all living within a clean environment not yet polluted by chemicals and acidity. To keep the body in this state, one could follow a relatively low-sugar, low-carb diet and avoid carcinogens, like pesticides, and foods filled with hormones and antibiotics, or fried in omega 6 oils.

But few children and young adults do this, and the more one is exposed to excesses the greater the damage.

Here are how cells react to these damaging inputs.

Healthy cells have just the right amount of oxygen, the right amount of salt, and the right acid/alkaline Ph balance, and the body has a strong compass that keeps these levels on track.

If, for example, one ingests foods requiring great stomach acidity to break them down – hamburgers, fries and a soda – the intestines pull some of this acid into the blood stream, leaving it acidic. To get the blood back on track, bits of alkalinity are poached from other cells in the body by means of the *osmosis* interplay that continually takes place between the cells and the blood stream.

This fixes the blood. But though the blood has a corrected Ph level, the cells contributing alkalinity are left slightly acidic, and guess what? Cancer prefers acidity.

The same is true of salt. Our bodies are quite saline, close to the composition of sea water (the source of life on Earth). Hence one should ingest sea salt with food, as besides salt, sea salt has 90 other trace elements the body craves.

So, if one uses refined salt stripped of trace elements, then like Ph disequilibrium, the cells begin to cannibalize themselves pushing their own stores of trace elements back out to the blood stream. This restores the blood's saline composition, but the depleted cells suffer a form of mineral dehydration, which weakens them, and exposes them to viral attack.

Besides these dietary imbalances, external chemicals ingested or breathed into the body also need to be neutralized within the blood stream. The kidneys, liver and sweat glands do much of the scrubbing, but circulating chemicals are also pulled into the cells to help clear the blood. Chemical deposits result in a further acidic condition inside of the cells, which in turn, squeezes out some of the cell's supply of oxygen.

And guess what? Cancer hates oxygen.

And so, as you can expect, with healthy cells, many years of abuse will simply wear them down. Less abuse leads to lower levels of vulnerability. Hence cancer prevention starts in one's early years into one's 30's, 40's, 50's and beyond. Keep as clean as possible.

Most people do not know that the intake of sugar and simple carbs, along with the intake of omega-6 oils, greatly impinges the immune system.

Sugar and carbs require insulin activation for cells to absorb the incoming glucose. Effectively, this insulin spike becomes an internal stress episode. Stress of any kind results in a cortisol "stand down" order being broadcast to the immune cells, so that all energy can be directed at resolving the stress intrusion. In this case the stress trigger is sugar, in other cases it might be running from a barking dog, etc.

People with diabetes – slow glucose metabolism - experience even longer durations of stress, and hence their immune systems are muted for extended periods when dealing with sugar spikes. Viruses have a field day, unopposed. The solution is to avoid sugar and simple carb intake.

Omega-6 oils used by many fast food outlets trigger high levels of standing inflammation throughout the body, including the lungs. One of the outcomes of Covid-19 is something called a *Cytokine Storm*, the creation of too much inflammation in the lungs. If your lungs are already inundated with inflammation due to Omega-6, then the virus just piles on even greater levels, blocking the respiratory flow between the lungs and the blood stream.

Overall, stay away from fast food, and religiously use olive oil and garlic (anti-inflammatories) as cuisine staples.

One's weight is a reflection of one's diet. By avoiding sugars and carbs, one keeps the weight down, and eliminates the insulin stress episodes, allowing the immune response to keep its focus on invading antigens (viruses, bacteria, funguses & parasites).

A study published May 1 2020 in the journal Cell Metabolism found that people with diabetes who keep their blood sugar levels in a tighter range were much less likely to have a severe Covid-19 disease course than those with more fluctuations in their blood sugar levels.

One more thing, exercise. One's cells are serviced by two vessel systems – blood and lymph. Cells live inside a liquid bubble that in turn is touched by blood and lymph capillaries. In order to supply the cells, these vessel systems need to move red blood and lymph fluids along in order to reach the cells. The heart moves the blood, and bodily movement moves the lymph. Get as much exercise as possible to fine tune these supply lines.

Related to exercise, is the fact that vessels lose elasticity as one ages, which makes the heart work harder. A supplement made from red grape skins called Resveratrol (see appendix), helps to keep vessels supple. The benefit of Resveratrol is sometimes referred to as "The French red wine effect", because the French who drink red wine daily have fewer heart disease issues.

Magnesium also works to keep ones blood vessels supple (described in more detail later).

Phase 2
Assaulted Cells

No matter what we do, all of us are susceptible to viral attacks at any age. It is just a question of how vulnerable, and the severity.

Once viruses enter the blood stream, they seek to penetrate cells where they live off of a host cell and reproduce. And once inside a cell, besides reproducing, an active virus can switch healthy cells cancerous during cell division. And so, the next line of defense against cancer involves anything that blunts viral attacks.

2a. Blood Antiseptics

Many are not aware that the blood stream contains antiseptics that sicken viruses, substances like iodine and zinc. Viruses might get into the bloodstream but become weak or even killed by the antiseptics, never getting as far as penetrating cells so that they can reproduce. Feeble viruses floating around in the bloodstream is not infection.

True viral infection means that viruses have penetrated cells and have worked their way to cell nucleuses. Once getting into the nucleus, a single virus divides into 20,000 offspring viruses, with all of the fledgling viruses feeding off of the cell. Once the 20,000 are ready, they leave that cell looking for new territory to invade (shedding). The 20,000 each produce 20,000 more viruses, and quite suddenly we have 400,000,000 infected cells.

The first line of defense are these blood antiseptics that repel viruses while still in the blood stream - before they have the chance to penetrate cells. Three key antiseptics are iodine, zinc and apple cider vinegar, which one can take as supplements.

> i) **Iodine** is especially important with breast tissue. Because of the menstrual cycle, cell division and programmed cell death oscillate with the monthly cycle. During this time, viruses lurking in the breast tissue seek to penetrate cells. Once cells are penetrated and dividing, the door is open to create an offspring breast cell now switched cancerous.
>
> As reported by Dr. Russel Blaylock "Recent studies have found 100 percent incidence of cytomegalovirus (a herpes strain) in breast cancer tumors, and 94 percent incidence in the lymph nodes draining these cancers." See research at: *link. springer.com/article/10.1007/s12094-019-02164-1*
>
> Woman carry large concentrations of Iodine in their thyroid gland, their breast tissue and in their ovaries for this very antiseptic purpose. It has been found that woman with low Iodine levels develop breast cancer at much higher rates. Iodine deficiency is often tied to thyroid issues, so both thyroid hormonal output and Iodine levels need to be measured by your doctor.
>
> The question becomes how much Iodine should be added via supplementation. The Japanese, with

their seaweed staple, have 10 to 20 times more Iodine than western woman, and they experience fewer outbreaks of breast cancer, so speak to a naturopathic doctor about this consideration.

ii) **Zinc** too, is an antiseptic, and it became famous during Covid-19 as an agent that blunted the Coronavirus. But it hurts all viruses, so a daily supplement is merited, especially for men, as men's prostate glands use zinc the way woman's breast tissue uses Iodine.

iii) **Apple Cider Vinegar** has been used from Greek times onward as an external disinfectant for wounds, but it can be ingested as food, and distributed amongst the bodies blood supply, adding one more antiseptic to the mix. It is available in pill and gummy form.

Take your antiseptic boosts daily to keep viruses weak.

2b. - Cell Wall defenses & Vitamin provisions

Many do not realize that oxygen is problematic once inside the body. Skin and lung cells tolerate direct exposure to oxygen, but internal cells cannot. What does this mean? Just as iron exposed to oxygen rusts, and a cut apple turns brown, one's internal cells can effectively be burnt by oxygen. To counter this, the internal cells coat themselves with a chemical shield made up of antioxidant molecules. Oxygen then enters the cell via specialized oxygen-proof receptor portals sitting on the cell wall.

i) **Vitamin C** - The most famous antioxidant is Vitamin C, but there are many others, including berries and green tea. Because vitamin C is water soluble, it gets flushed out by the kidneys, and needs to be replenished daily to maintain an adequate level. The standard dose is 500 mg twice a day, but in the presence of a viral attack, larger dosses are called for. Keep the cell walls protected from oxidative stress, and let the cells concentrate on repelling viruses.

ii) **Vitamin D3** – Besides antioxidants, one needs to maintain a certain level of Vitamin D3 in the cells. Vitamin D3 is really a hormone created by the body when skin is exposed to the sun. This hormone keeps every cell on its toes, allowing cells to fully express the various operational blueprints sitting within the cell's DNA – e.g. formulas specifying how to repel viruses; formulas governing immune cell alertness, formulas keeping inflammation in check.

Low D3 makes cells sluggish. Very low D3 can be felt as depression if the brain cells are not fully provisioned with D3. So, if cells are to stay vigilant in resisting viral penetration, they need proper D3 to stay the course.

D3 is usually lower in the cooler seasons with reduced sunlight, the very season where viruses flourish. D3 is reduced further based upon dark skin color. 50% of Covid-19 deaths in America were Americans of color; and though other factors were in play, these people needed more supplementation. D3 is fat soluble, meaning that the body can store reserves of it. To keep the reserves replenished, most people need to take D3 daily in 5,000 – 7,000 units based upon skin color. A blood test reveals your level, indicating your dosage needs. Note: take D3, not D2 supplements.

The National Institute of Health says this: *Vitamin D has many roles in the body, including modulation of cell growth, neuromuscular and immune function, and reduction of inflammation. Many genes encoding proteins that regulate cell proliferation, differentiation, and apoptosis are modulated in part by vitamin D. Many cells have vitamin D receptors.*

Dr. JoAnn Manson, Professor at Harvard Medical says this: *Vitamin D may be relevant to the risk of developing Covid-19 as well as affecting the severity of the disease. Vitamin D not only boosts the immune system but lowers inflammation, which mitigates the respiratory response during Covid-19, including damaging cytokine storms.*

iii) Magnesium

Magnesium is used throughout the body in hundreds of ways. Here we will look at just a few of its attributes.

- *Mitochondria Need Magnesium*

    Mitochondria are little organisms that live inside of your cells. Their job is to take in nutrients, and combine these with the oxygen to generate electrical charges to power the cells – organic "power plants", if you will.

    To achieve this, your tiny mitochondria convert both glucose and ketone nutrient packets into energy, but they need magnesium to achieve this.

    If the mitochondria are happy, then they quickly extract nutrients from the blood stream and keep your energy level high.

    When mitochondria lack magnesium they are slow to absorb glucose sugars, so that excess sugar simply circulates 'round and 'round in the blood stream, *giving cancer time to absorb it. A diabetic pattern.*

Because magnesium speeds up the "micro" metabolism of sugars, as a bi product, it effectively dampens type II diabetes.

Finally, magnesium increases the water levels in your intestinal system, so that your bowel movements stay balanced.

Too little magnesium leads to constipation, too much magnesium leads to diarrhea. Based upon experience, your magnesium dosage can be finetuned to find the right level for your system.

Trial and error are the best approaches, as standing magnesium levels can only be tested in the blood stream, and these tests do not measure absorption by the cells.

- *Magnesium Reserves Dwindle with Age*

    As said, magnesium stands important to your wellbeing, and as one ages past age 30, the level of supplementation needs increase, towards 300 + mg per day for women older than 50. But again, fine tune the dosage with your naturopath or nutritionist.

iv) CoQ10/PQQ

One more supplement to take to blunt viruses is a combination of CoQ10 and PQQ, two enzymes needed by the mitochondria to do their energy-producing job. Certain cells, like heart cells, have thousands of mitochondria living in each cell. Give the mitochondria what they need in order to keep the cells robust, able to resist viruses. A combined CoQ10/PQQ supplement is listed in the appendix.

Phase 3
Infected

Even with adequate levels of antiseptics and cell vitamin enhancement, no one can prevent viral infection throughout one's life. These infections start with the simple cold, to the flu, to Covid-19, to Chicken Pox, to Measles, to Herpes, to HPV and HIV.

Once infected, the body calls up the immune system to come in and kill the antigen invaders. Hence, we want to provision the immune system (T-cells, Natural Killer Cells, etc.) with things that strengthen their resolve. Vitamins, sleep and a detoxed system allow the immune agents to do their best. Let's start with vitamin supplements, then move on to sleep, closing with detoxing.

3a. – Immune Cell Support - Supplements

Four supplements support and amplify the specialized cells of the immune system.

i) **Beta Glucan** - The first is *Beta Glucan*, a vitamin found in many foods, particularly in oats, but you can augment digested Beta Glucan with pills to ensure an adequate level persists. Naturopathic practitioners recommend taking Beta Glucan pills every other day, but daily once you are under attack. Like vitamin C, Beta Glucan is water soluble, so excesses are washed out daily.

ii) **Red Reishi Mushroom** - The second is *Red Reishi Mushroom* extract. This can be purchased in pill form. Organic molecules from this mushroom stimulate the immune cells to become more aggressive in seeking out invading antigens.

iii) **Vitamin A** – A third vitamin needed to kill off viruses is *Vitamin A*. Vitamin A fuels immune cells, especially in the respiratory track – throat/lungs. If getting a sore throat, a cough, or tightness in the chest (all Covid-19 symptoms), take vitamin A only for a few days, as A is fat soluble, easily stored.

Doctor Brownstein, a research & clinical MD reports: To treat acute viral infections in healthy adults, I recommend 100,000 IU of vitamin A per day along with 50,000 IU of vitamin D3, both for four days.

iv) **Astragalus**

Astragalus is a plant extract that supports the production of lymphocytes, immune cells that kill viruses. As reported by Doctor Blaylock:

People with serious Covid-19 illness have very low counts of lymphocytes. Take a 2,000 mg capsule of Astragalus daily.

3b. - Sleep & Salt Baths

A further provision is sleep. During the day, while in an active awake state, your *sympathetic* nervous system dominates, operating your motor functions and your sensory activity. The immune system is significantly lowered during the day to funnel energy to the physical operation of the body. Once asleep, your *para-sympathetic* system kicks in, triggering deeper levels of digestion, cellular repair and focused immune system action against viruses and cancer tumors. This is why most fevers are broken at night.

Once you are truly infected by any virus or tumor outbreak, get as much sleep as your body calls for. Taking a sea salt bath before bedtime helps to switch from sympathetic to para-sympathetic dominance, allowing the immune system to gear up for the night.

The baths also elevate your temperature, helping to stimulate the immune cells into action, the way fevers do.

And, the salt itself allows the skin to absorb any trace minerals still lacking in the blood stream, lacking after digested sources.

Salt supplies are delivered to your door, so add this protocol into your nightly regimen.

3c. Detoxing

Foreign chemicals in the body hurt all cells, but the "combat ready" immune cells get it the worst, as they need to be nimble and aggressive. In the past 100 years over 1,000 toxic chemicals have been introduced into our food and environment.

It is noted that chemotherapy chemicals in particular weigh heavily on the system. Not only do the chemo mixtures poison every cell in the body, but their chemical makeup is acidic, squeezing oxygen out of the cells (described shortly).

Fighting off viruses in any kind of polluted state is like washing dishes in dirty water.

So how does one clean their system after a lifetime of chemical accumulation? Through three steps: Liver Detox, Fat Cell Detox and Homeopathic Detox. But be advised, the only two difficult aspects of Naturopathic rehabilitation comprise Detoxing and Diet. We cover Diet later. For now, let's take the Detox procedures in order.

i) Liver Detox

Besides your kidneys and sweat glands, the main engine for detoxing the body is the liver. Every drop of blood circulating the body passes through the liver every 20 minutes. Impurities in the blood are absorbed by the sponge-like tissue of the liver. And once isolated from the blood, impurities leach through the liver and flow into the gall bladder to be emptied into your intestinal track for excretion.

After many decades of performing this job 24/7, the liver loses efficiency as residual impurities become trapped amongst the liver tissue.

The liver itself needs a cleaning.

It may take a few weeks, but the liver can pretty much clean itself out if not stressed by things like alcohol, caffeine, nicotine, drugs, and difficult-to-process food nutrients. Plus, stimulants can help the liver along to release even deeper, residual deposits.

Naturopathic doctors, Nutritional specialists, and Eastern practitioners all offer herbal stimulants that trigger the release of embedded toxins from the liver. You'll need to find one to work with.

For those "addicted" to alcohol, caffeine and nicotine, the battle is tougher, as these practices need to be broken before also adding the cleanse supplement. This could take additional weeks.

For a few days whenever going "cold turkey", released toxins temporarily flow through the blood stream, and one feels woozy, with a sustained headache. Do not give in. Drink plenty of water. Once the bulk of hidden toxins clears, one feels clarity and new energy.

At this point, thankfully, Step 1 of detoxing is complete, and you will be very pleased with the result.

ii) Fat Cell Detox

Step 2 – fat cell detox – takes longer. Beside the liver, fat cells are used by the body to warehouse various excesses floating around the blood stream – particularly fat triglycerides and unwanted toxins.

One has a fixed amount of fat cells distributed throughout the body, and to handle excesses, each cell expands like a balloon. And as anyone trying to lose weight knows, these balloons do not empty easily.

Later, in *Phase 5 – Tumor Formed*, we will cover fat in more detail, but the process of shrinking fat cells starts by eliminating sugars and carbohydrates from your diet, forcing the body to call out its own fat reserves for its moment-by-moment energy supply. The new energy supply will be in the form of ketone packets, which replace glucose sugar packets. As said, more detail to come.

Based upon your fat reserves, and by following a vegetable-led ketone diet, it may take as little as 6 weeks to as long as a year to reach your baseline, near-zero-fat weight. Once that weight is reached, rather than harvesting one's remaining fat, outside fat sources, like chicken and fish, are re-introduced. Details coming up shortly.

But for now, *Step 2 – Fat Detox* via weight loss is complete, and you will feel and look "marvelous".

iii) Homeopathic Detox

This leads us to an even deeper, body-wide detox, called "homeopathic detox". The Homeopathic approach is scoffed at by many but start by understanding it before ignoring the claimed benefits.

> The premise of Homeopathic Detox is that "like" materials attract each other. Bits of mercury are attracted to other bits of mercury, the way the earth and moon pull at each other.
>
> But the nuance of Homeopathic treatment utilizes an electromagnetic image of mercury that can be imprinted in water (like an electromagnetic image of sound imprinted on a CD), and this water, though not holding real mercury, still pulls on hidden deposits of physical mercury buried within one's structural cells. The deep mercury is dislodged and swept out by the liver and kidney organs.

Homeopathic Detox is offered by Biological Dentists, who test and treat the patient for as many as 500 hidden carcinogens. Find such a practitioner in your area.

After the Liver, Fat Cell and Homeopathic Detox steps are complete, you have restored your internal chemistry to near childhood levels of cleanliness. Your immune system will hum!

Phase 4
Converted

The fourth phase of cancer development is the point where normal cells are switched cancerous.

How does this happen?

4a. Conventional Theory

This topic is controversial. Conventional medicine does not claim to know the answer (see the Defeating Breast Cancer book for the debates coming out of conventional medicine). Overall, the conventional line of thought is as follows:

Mainstream medicine theories claim cancer happens when a cell's DNA *mutates in a spontaneous manner during cell division*, but this constitutes naïvete in our opinion. Too many thousands of DNA genes would have to mutate, all in perfect harmony, for the new cancer cell to operate cohesively. In other words, the *various thousands of genes and the vast numbers of switch-setting combinations among chromosome strands would require perfect synchronization to keep the emerging cell's biochemical factory operating.*

Most true mutations result in cell death as the isolated mutation falls out of step with the vast DNA matrix operating the cell.

4b. Understanding DNA Switches

The amount of DNA inside a cell can overwhelm your comprehension. Some 20,000 different genes reside, with each gene switched on and off (*expressed*) via millions of molecular switch combinations. These switches are like the brail spindle on a player piano activating piano keys.

Certain switches activate sets of genes that determine each cell's assigned role in the body ("you're a skin cell").

Other gene switches happen in real time as the cell spars with oxygen depletion, toxin and stimulant absorption, hormonal commands, or viral invasions.

Consider this description coming out of the University of Washington in 2012 on the depth of switches resident within your DNA:

> *The locations of millions of DNA 'switches' that dictate how, when, and where in the body different genes turn on and off have been identified by a team of researchers at the University of Washington in Seattle. Genes make up only 2 percent of the human genome and were easy to spot, but the on/off switches controlling those genes were encrypted within the remaining 98 percent of the genome. Without these switches, called regulatory DNA, genes are inert.*

4c. Cancer Uniformity Across the Population

More so, in the face of the above, even if *spontaneous, synchronized mutations across DNA strands* could even occur in a single cell, they would have to occur over and over again in the exact manner across the entire human population to result in, for instance, a particular breast cancer type called *estrogen sensitive cancer* that 70 percent of breast cancer patients contract.

For anyone to intellectually hold onto *universally identical mass mutations happening "spontaneously" among all beings across the vast human species* - as the root cause of estrogen sensitive breast cancer - constitutes conceptual folly in our opinion.

Also, we found the following statement buried inside The American Cancer Society's website listed under "Viruses" but not under "Cancers."

> *"Viruses are very small organisms; most can't even be seen with an ordinary microscope. They are made up of a small group of genes in the form of DNA or RNA surrounded by a protein coating.*
>
> *Viruses need to enter a living cell and 'hijack' the cell's machinery to reproduce and make more viruses. Some viruses do this by inserting their own DNA (or RNA) into that of the host cell. When the DNA or RNA affects the host cell's genes, it may push the cell toward becoming cancer."*

And so, where does this lead us?

4d. The Viral Theory

The counter-theory to spontaneous mutation, is viral interference with DNA switch settings during the copy step of cell division.

Alternative switch options are readily available in the DNA library, so when a cell is switched to one of these other options, alternative yet proven DNA blueprints are used for the offspring cancer cell to stay alive. It is still a Breast

Cell, but now it has been switched to operate as a cancerous Breast Cell.

Ok, what can be done with these unsuitably switched cells?

4e. Putting Cancer to Sleep

Research coming out of Purdue University, headed by Doctors James and Dorothy Morre, found differences on the cell walls of normal versus cancerous cells. Specifically, the cell receptors (antennas) that listen for the hormonal signals broadcast throughout the body, operated differently.

With normal cells, the receptor "hears" both divide and die signals, but the cancer receptor only "hears" divide signals. Hence cancer cells never contemplate dying, only division.

Looking deeper, the researchers isolated the ENOX gene as the one creating this receptor and found two switch settings: An ENOX1 switch which grows a receptor able to hear both divide and die impulses, and an ENOX2 switch which grows a receptor that only records divide impulses.

Because cancer cells are switched ENOX2, they never hear hormonal commands telling them to die. What can be done with this insight?

Well, if the ENOX2 receptor could be "muzzled" or "plugged", then the cancer cell would cease receiving divide signals, and would lay dormant until dying of inactivity or through immune attacks.

A compound that plugs the ENOX2 receptor was found in green tea. To make this solution practical, the researches developed a green tea pill with the equivalent of 16 cups of tea per pill (see Capsol-T in the appendix).

They next performed clinical tests and had excellent results with over 90% of the participants.

So, buy these pills! One for daytime use, and a time release version for night.

Also, because cancerous switching starts with viruses, please visit a vivid U.K. animated documentary on viruses and the cell battleground, here:

http://www.dailymotion.com/video/x1f26gz_bbc-our-secret-universe-the-hidden-life-of-the-cell-720p-hdtv_tech

Phase 5
Tumor Formed

The most important things to know about cancer tumors are how difficult they are to detect and how long they need to be growing to become detectable.

The time frames vary, but 6 to 10 years to be visible on a mammogram is a good estimate. At that point, the tumor consists of 500 million cells, and it is still tiny. More developed tumors have billions of cells.

Besides seeing a tumor, Oncologists can detect evidence of cancer via blood tests that look for "markers". Markers are specific chemicals released by each type of cancer into the blood stream. For example, Colon Cancer markers differ from Breast Cancer markers. But even here, around 2 million cancer cells are needed for the markers to be measurable.

Until its later stages cancer moves slowly, providing time to counter it before it becomes dominant, able to metastasize. And so, how does one counter developing cancer tumors?

First, there are the conventional steps of surgery, radiation and chemotherapy which deliver a direct assault on the tumors, though with much collateral damage to the body. Plus, these invasive steps do nothing to rehabilitate the body, avoiding further breakouts down the line. But these one-sided invasive choices are often selected, as the patient is unaware of Naturopathic possibilities.

Second, are the Naturopathic steps, designed to take the tumor out of its comfort zone by depriving it of nutrients, by infiltrating it with substances that slow and arrest its cell division trajectory, and by increasing the resolve of the immune system.

Third, some woman develop a condition called Dense Breast Tissue, which makes them four times more likely to develop breast cancer. Dense Breast tissue provides a breeding ground for cancer. One needs to understand this phenomenon, and take offsetting countermeasures.

We start with Diet, the most difficult-to-stick-to aspect of Naturopathic rehabilitation, and then cover the easy-to-implement infiltration measures, and finally discuss Dense Breast Tissue, as well as frameworks on radiation and chemotherapy.

5a. Glucose Diets

Most readers have heard that sugar is closely connected to cancer. Actually, cancer requires sixteen times more sugar than normal cells.

But there is something else.

Healthy cells create energy *aerobically* by combining oxygen and sugar, called *oxidation*, similar to burning logs on a fire, whereas cancer cells hide from oxygen and instead create their energy *anaerobically* by *fermenting* large quantities of sugar as does a whisky still.

Cancer cells require sixteen times as much sugar than normal cells to achieve fermentation.

With cancer this hungry for sugar, the diet centerpiece for blunting cancer seeks to provide the body with just enough energy for healthy cells while leaving cancer tumors high and dry. "Just enough" comes in the form of the carbohydrates found in vegetables.

The day you start with a sugar-restrictive diet is the day the cancer cells begin to go hungry. As the weeks go by, and the body's hidden sugar reserves dwindle, tumor cells slowly die of starvation.

Sugar (glucose), comes in the form of direct sugars (candy, soda, alcohol, fruit) and indirect sugars made from carbohydrates (bread, pasta, potatoes, rice). Eliminating these may be difficult for you, but the cancer will hate it, and your normal cells will love it.

Additionally, there is a natural supplement called "Gloucose Reduce" that flattens sugar spikes (see appendix).

5b. Ketone Diets

Actually, the cells do fine without all that sugar. Using fats and proteins, your liver creates energy packets called "ketones", and healthy cells can digest ketones, *but cancer cannot.*

This fuel switch – from heavy sugars to ketones – isolates the cancer.

Realize this … our bodies were designed for ketone metabolism in the first place.

Sugar cane was only discovered in the Americas 500 years ago, and prior diets carried no direct sugars, only fruit sugars and derived sugars from carbohydrates. And even carbohydrates – wheat, oats, etc., are really only 4,000 years old. And once, fruit was very rare.

Before that we were paleo people – fats, proteins, nuts and root vegetables.

Modern diets are sugar dominated, benefiting cancer. So, in fighting cancer, one needs to cut out direct sugars and sugar-generating carbohydrates all together.

This gets you back to a more natural state which relies upon a greater use of animal fats, proteins and oils.

In doing so, your body will naturally switch back to creating ketone energy packets as its main energy source.

5c. Here is how ketone energy works.

You may have heard of ketones in both paleo and ketone diets. Ketones are a separate energy source from glucose sugar - made from fat rather than from sugars and carbohydrates.

But as long as there is plenty of sugar, the body holds off from making ketones. Conversely, when sugar is absent in the blood stream, and the cells are hungry, your fat cells receive hormone signals to release stored triglycerides, a human fat molecule.

The liver converts the triglycerides into ketones and passes these along to the cells as a fuel packet.

Going ketonic means replacing glucose packets with these ketone packets. The secret: ketones don't work with cancer cells. Here's why.

5d. The Mitochondria

As mentioned, Mitochondria are the little organisms living in our cells that generate energy. Each cell's Mitochondria convert incoming nutrients into the electrical energy that powers the cell's biochemistry.

As they oxidize nutrients, Mitochondria generate an electrically charged molecule, called STP, that travels inside the cell, like a floating battery.

Ketones can be metabolized by these healthy mitochondria, whereas cancer mitochondria are inactive, which is why Cancer can only ferment glucose, not able to oxidize ketone nutrients.

I will say it again:

Feeding the body via ketones isolates the cancer from its sugar supply.

5e. Smooth Energy with Ketones

Ketones offer another advantage; they provide an even supply of energy throughout the day – no hunger spikes.

Consistency is achieved by your kidneys, which regulate ketone volumes, purging excess ketone levels. This ensures no ups and downs, and one experiences a calmer mental and emotional state as the ketones are metabolized.

However, too much fat intake can make the liver make too many ketones, which can stress out the kidneys, so unlike the Atkins diet, which allows unlimited fat intake, moderation is called for with true ketonic diets.

5f. Ketone Meals

You can find cuisine guidance on various web sites for ketone-led meals, so we will only say this at the ROADMAP level.

There is Ketone, and then there is "Super Ketone". Initially when shedding fat reserves, to seriously impinge tumors, super ketone is required. With super ketone, no animal meats are added to the diet. You stick to vegetables and salads, with some nuts and olive oil to add bits of oil. You want to harvest the body's stored fat and keep energy supplies lean.

Once at your naturally lean weight, add chicken and fish three times a week. Admittedly, this is a hard row to hoe, but things fall into place one month into the new lifestyle.

Note on sugar: Many doctors point out that one's brain needs glucose, as a way of dismissing ketones. The missed point is that even with ketonic diets, glucose is still present, but only at the level needed by healthy cells, not at the 16x level cancer craves. Excess sugar also corrupts your vascular system and you skin, called glycation. Stay focused on sugar.

5g. Infiltrate the Tumors

Now that you are starving the tumors, you inflict greater damage. You can disorient them and destabilize their division rate trajectory. We will discuss four ways of infiltrating tumors.

i) Baking Soda

Baking soda is fully alkaline, something that can neutralize the acidic nature of cancer cells. But how to get it into the tumor?

A well-practiced solution is to mix baking soda into honey and ingest this. The tumor greedily ingests the sugar-laden honey and, in doing so, intolerable amounts of the alkaline baking soda penetrate the tumor cells, neutralizing the cancer's acidity, its comfort zone.

The preparation for the honey-baking soda follows:

Combine half a cup of honey and half a cup of baking soda in a glass.

- Place the glass in a stovetop pan with heated water and stir for eight minutes.
- Ingest a tablespoon each day.

ii) CBD infused with Frankincense

Our second infiltration technique involves CBD Oil derived from hemp plants, infused with frankincense.

Frankincense is an *essential* oil that confuses cancer cells over whether or not to divide. Frankincense inhibits the division trigger.

To get the cancer cells to ingest the frankincense, the frankincense is mixed into the CBD hemp oil by a Colorado firm called *Bluebird Botanicals* (see appendix). Here is how it works.

CBD molecules happen to have receptors that match up with cancer cell receptors so that by ingesting CBD, you effectively coat the cancer tumor with hemp oil.

CBD oil stuck onto cancer cell walls acts like an antibody, attracting immune cells.

By mixing in some frankincense with the hemp oil, you have delivered a double blow to the tumor. The CBD oil first serves as a beacon to lure immune cells to check out the tumor, and second, through osmosis, the tumor absorbs the unwanted frankincense right into its gut.

CBD Oil + Frankincense is an liquid oil that you put under your tongue daily.

iii) Saffron

The spice saffron offers another powerful anti-cancer ingredient. Life Extension Magazine says this about saffron:

> *"The first step in cancer development is some kind of trigger that initiates malignant transformation. This may be an environmental toxin, a stray oxygen radical, or invasion with certain viruses. Saffron components have been shown to help prevent outbreaks caused by each of these triggers.*
>
> *Saffron extracts have also been shown to potently prevent DNA damage caused by free radicals, radiation, and inflammation, thereby reducing the risk of new cancer formation.*
>
> *Once a cell has been triggered to become malignant, it then proliferates, or reproduces rapidly and without normal controls, to produce a developing tumor.*

> *Studies show that saffron is able to suppress — and in some cases reverse — the proliferation of certain human cancer cells in culture.*
>
> *For example, one compelling study found that breast cancer cells treated with saffron extract displayed significant reductions in proliferation, to as low as 2.8% of the rate seen in untreated cells."*

With scientific data like the above, one should certainly add a simple-to-take saffron pill to one's supplement list.

iv) Intravenous Vitamin C

Some alternative-therapy practitioners advocate intravenous injections of vitamin C. The direct injection of the vitamin prevents the digestive tract from compromising the C molecule.

Proponents claim that the body converts concentrated C into substances that affect the anaerobic-fermenting-of-sugar mechanism that rogue cancer cells depend upon.

The derived compound contains H_2O_2 (hydrogen peroxide), which, in turn, floods cancer cells with unwanted oxygen.

Because you need to have an IV installed, a medical professional needs to be involved. Intravenous vitamin "C" should be considered as one more weapon for your arsenal, especially with advanced cancer situations.

5h. Dense Breast Tissue

So, what do they mean by "dense breast tissue"? The Susan G Kommen ™ web site explains:

> "Breast density is not a measure of how the breasts feel, but rather how the breasts look on a mammogram.
>
> High-breast density means there is a greater amount of breast connective tissue as compared to fat.
>
> Low-breast density means there is a greater amount of fat as compared to breast and connective tissue."

This "connective tissue" is a fibrous substance that holds the breast organ intact. But it also contains a type of scar tissue caused by the menstrual cycle. The "Wise GEEK" web site explains scar tissue:

> "Internal scar tissue can be formed by various causes including repetitive usage. The healing process will begin by forming fibroses tissue around the injury, forming a web that protects it from further harm.
>
> During this stage, the injured cells turn into adhesions, which are basically dead cells. As the area heals, the adhesions that were present will develop into permanent scar tissue."

In other words, fibrosis of the breast includes scar fibers resulting from the monthly wear and tear of the menstrual cycle. As breast cells divide and die each month leftover strands of scar fiber build up over decades.

This cluttered tissue becomes a breeding ground for viruses, and should cancer be triggered, it can hide from the immune system inside the dense web.

But what can be done?

Two supplements were found that break down scar tissue in the breast, and probably elsewhere in the body.

i) Evening Primrose Oil

Primrose oil is made from Prim Rose flowers. The flowers open at dusk and close with morning light, which is where the name *Evening* Prim Rose comes from.

Prim Rose Oil contains fatty acids that contribute in revitalizing breast cells struggling within the confines of all of those stringy fibers inside the breast. The oil apparently also works to alleviate forms of arthritis, again by revitalizing the good tissue lost within the arthritic area.

See appendix for a Primrose recommendation.

ii) Serraflazyme

Before describing serraflazyme, we will describe enzymes.

In general, *enzymes* are internally created chemicals made by the body designed to cause specific bio-chemical reactions to take place.

Enzymes are not to be confused with *hormones*, chemical triggers operating at a higher level directing *cellular behavior*. Instead each enzyme has a functional job.

The body make thousands of enzymes for various functional purposes, and the job of serraflazyme is to break-down scar tissue. Because scar tissue is an element of dense breast tissue, we like serraflazyme.

But here is a most telling piece of information.

Once in one's 30's, the body stops making adequate levels of serraflazyme. In younger years, scar tissue is removed from the body once the tissue area heals. But in later years, scar tissue remains amongst the living tissue for the rest of your life.

This is why one "lives" with one's injuries forever, even after healing.

In the case of scar tissue formed in the breast during menstrual cycles, each monthly cycle in your 30's leaves leftover scar tissue behind. And this continues until menopause, a 15 to 20 year build up needing to be broken down.

But there is more to this as the Susan B Kommen site explained.

If you have large breasts with a lot of fat, then the cumulative scar density is minor, as the fat cells can still provide blood and lymph pathways throughout the breast organ.

However, with smaller breasts, the scar density dominates, and blood and lymph support gets stifled.

As said, this opens the door to invading viruses that, left unchecked, can trigger a cancer switch-over during cell division. This is why, women with "dense breast tissue" have four times the chance of a cancer outbreak.

Luckily, research in the 1990s by a Doctor Lee isolated the serraflazyme enzyme, and now it is available in pill form.

At some point in your 30's you should look into taking this as a preventative measure.

See appendix for a recommendation.

iii) Radiation and Chemotherapy

Besides surgery, Conventional Medicine uses both radiation and chemotherapy to sicken cancer tumors. These therapies are outlined next.

5j. Radiation

Once tumors become visible on mammograms, radiation is often used to kill the cancer cells. The American Cancer Society describes the use of radiation to treat breast cancers as follows.

> Short term - If you have radiation to the breast, it can cause side effects such as skin irritation, dryness, color changes, soreness and swelling. Breast soreness, color changes, and fluid build-up will most likely go away a month or two after you finish radiation therapy.
>
> Long term - Radiation therapy may cause long-term changes in the breast. Your skin may be slightly darker, and pores may be larger and more noticeable. The skin may be more or less sensitive and feel thicker and firmer than it was before treatment. Sometimes the size of your breast changes.
>
> In rare cases, radiation therapy may weaken the ribs, which could lead to a fracture. Radiation can also affect the heart, cause hardening of the arteries (which

can make you more likely to have a heart attack later on), heart valve damage, or irregular heartbeats.

Getting radiation to the breast can sometimes cause an inflammation of the lungs, which is called radiation pneumonitis. Radiation to the breast can sometimes damage some of the nerves to the arm.

So yes, radiation kills cancer cells, but agree to it with your eyes open. It will be described to you primarily from the optic of improved five-year survival statistics, with less emphasis on collateral damage, and no claims of any 5 to 20-year implications. Be mindful that once treated with radiation, should a cancer re-occurrence happen, the tissue impacted cannot be re-treated with radiation a second time.

Radiation follows a lumpectomy to kill off cancer cells still present in the breast and lymph nodes. Generally, a lumpectomy without radiation results in a cancer re-occurrence 25% of the time, whereas a lumpectomy with radiation results in a cancer re-occurrence 12.5% of the time. Mastectomies require no radiation (nothing to radiate) and re-occurrence falls to the single digits.

5k. Chemotherapy

With more advanced cases of Breast Cancer, chemotherapy is often used to attack both the visible and invisible outcroppings of the cancer.

Chemotherapy started from experiments with mustard gas stockpiles left over from World War I. Researchers turned the mustard agent into a poison that could be infused into the bloodstream. The idea started and remains to take advantage of cancer's very active metabolism and rapid cell division rates to absorb poison more aggressively than other cells.

Every cell in the body is poisoned with the cancer cells getting it the worst. The poison, though, seriously harms any normal cell that also has fairly high metabolism and cell division rates. These include hair, bone marrow, stomach, and intestine cells.

The punishment these innocent cells endure during chemotherapy results in the familiar side effects: hair loss, lowered blood counts, nausea, fatigue, and infections. Not only does chemotherapy weaken all cells but also the chemo drug itself is acidic causing an overall septic condition to settle in throughout the body.

The net result: cancer cells are killed, but with permanent weakening of the bone marrow, reduced ability to absorb essential nutrients, weakened immunity and emboldened tumors that may grow resistant to chemo ... all with nothing accomplished to prevent another bout of cancer to incubate at a future date.

Even if you agree to chemotherapy, one should use Naturopathic measures to bolster the body's internal abilities to counteract immediate and long term outbreaks of Breast Cancer. Outsourcing your treatment to drugs alone is an incomplete strategy.

One further issue with chemotherapy that may catch you by surprise is that doctors often order no supplements taken whatsoever, even things like vitamin C. They want to avoid unintended consequences at the bio-chemical level. Essentially, Chemotherapy is a "total war" election where collateral damage is acceptable.

An "organic" note: Chemotherapeutic drugs are often derived from plants, the way penicillin comes from a fungus, but the chemo is poisonous, the penicillin curative.

Phase 6
Aggression

Many have read that chronic inflammation pushes cancer tumors to grow at faster rates. In this chapter, we will dissect the "why" mystery, and suggest ways to shut down chronic inflammation.

6a. What is Inflammation?

Inflammation is the body's response to damage or irritation – such as a cut, a sprain, a mosquito bite or pollen particles reaching your lungs.

Once a disruption occurs, many bio-chemical and immune system components all jump in, forming the body's "massive" inflammatory response.

Collectively, inflammation agents …

i) *attack infection caused by invading viruses, bacteria, funguses, parasites and unwanted chemicals,*
ii) *dissolve damaged and dead cells,*
iii) *regulate blood supply at the trauma area, and*
iv) *trigger healing through stem cell activation and cell divisions that replace damaged tissue.*

That's quite the set of duties carried out by one's "inflammatory response", but inflammation can take on two modes of behavior in carrying out its mission.

6b. Acute versus Chronic Inflammation

What is called "Acute inflammation" lasts just long enough to heal a specific injury. Once healed, all of the inflammatory biochemical activity is shut down.

For example, your mosquito bite stops itching, or your swollen ankle calms down.

But if some form of irritant remains in the body, the inflammation response persists, never shutting down. This runaway situation is called *chronic* inflammation.

For example, if you are gluten intolerant, but eat gluten, your intestines will experience chronic inflammation.

Another example includes the endless discomfort of arthritis, where the body keeps attacking the arthritic deposits building up in the bone joints.

Other examples include the auto-immune diseases of lupus and crone's disease, where the body attacks itself as the enemy.

It is this type of chronic, on-going inflammation that drives cancer.

6c. Why does chronic inflammation drive cancer?

In general, inflammation triggers the bio-chemical activities needed for healing – things like stem cell conversions and rapid cell division rates... processes that shore up tissue reconstruction. So, what has all of this do with cancer?

Cancer tumors are your own cells, and so cancer itself may not trigger inflammation. But tumors can nevertheless cause stress amongst the normal cells that surround it.

Localized stress attracts neutrophils and macrophages which in turn create a pool of inflammation around the tumor.

And here is the kicker – besides stimulating local stem cells, inflammation stimulates cancer cells. Inflammation causes cancer cells to divide more aggressively.

This is why sonogram examinations are on the lookout for three things: rogue cell formations, dense breast tissue situations, and pockets of inflammation.

Ok, so how do we counter excessive inflammation build up when in fact, no tissue damage is in play?

A macro approach might be to use steroids, like prednisone, which shutter the whole immune system down. But that is far too debilitating.

Instead, here are five (5) naturopathic approaches.

i) **Antioxidants**

The first is to boost antioxidants so that overall, your cells are shielded from free radicals, lowering stress levels. Lowered stress levels relax the neutrophils, who back off from creating runaway inflammation.

Besides vitamin C, here are a few good antioxidant supplements and foods.

- Prim Rose Hips.
- Alpha-Lipoic Acid
- Curcumin
- Fish Oil
- Ginger
- Resveratrol
- Spirulina

And foods, such as:

- tomatoes
- olive oil
- green leafy vegetables, such as spinach and kale
- nuts like almonds and walnuts
- fruits such as strawberries and blueberries

All of these work at the biochemical level to protect the individual cells.

ii) **Copaiba Oil**

Second, beyond protecting cells, one can take Copaiba Oil to interrupt the stress-inflammation chain. Copaiba Oil has a molecule called Beta-caryophyllene that causes reduced stress levels at the cellular level.

Two drops of the oil can be added to your morning tea, plus Copaiba Oil can be applied on the skin above a tumor site, so that the Beta-caryophyllene gets to the inflamed area from within and without. A pill version is also available.

iii) Insulin Levels

A third driver to runaway inflammation is any persistent level of insulin in the blood stream. Insulin excess comes from the body's attempt to manage glucose sugar.

As explained in earlier chapters, elimination of sugars and carbs will curb this.

iv) Stress Levels

But there is a higher-level mechanism to stem inflammation, your nervous system. If you are all revved up, the body produces hormones like adrenalin and cortisol that implicitly signal "stress" to every cell in the body.

Therefore, the fourth driver to runaway inflammation is a persistent level of cortisol. Cortisol excess comes from heightened "fight-or-flight" situations in one's daily life, some you cannot avoid.

But you can tamper stress down if you are mindful of it. Take the nightly salt baths and work on calming your emotions down. These repetitive habits will create an on-going climate of rest.

The nervous system needs help, and the best relief comes from taking a B Complex vitamin daily (see appendix).

v) Toxins

Finally, toxins cause stress.

An earlier chapter described the impact of the over 1,000 toxic chemicals introduced into the environment since the 1800's. You can safely consider most of these to be irritants that trigger inflammation.

The answer to modern living calls for detoxing one's accumulated poisons, and to eat as healthy as possible going forward. These detox and diet measures were covered in other chapters. But for the purposes of this chapter on how inflammation drives cancer, one should keep in mind that toxins trigger inflammation.

vi) **The Chronic Inflammation Check List**

And so, the elimination of sugar, the adoption of antioxidants, the supplement Copaiba Oil, the policy of softened stress levels, and the detoxing of built-up irritants... will all go a long way in calming the body down, reducing persistent inflammation.

6d) Inflammatory Breast Cancer

There is one more topic one should be aware of, it is a condition called Inflammatory Breast Cancer, a rare form of cancer, usually surfacing in younger woman.

This specific condition stands separate from the general topic of chronic inflammation. Chronic inflammation affects all cancers; Inflammatory Breast Cancer is a specific type of cancer.

Here is the National Cancer Institute's summary on the Inflammatory Breast Cancer.

> *Inflammatory breast cancer is a rare and very aggressive disease in which cancer cells block lymph vessels in the skin of the breast. This type of breast cancer is called "inflammatory" because the breast often looks swollen and red, or inflamed.*
>
> *Inflammatory breast cancer accounts for 1 to 5 percent of all breast cancers diagnosed in the United*

> *States. Most inflammatory breast cancers develop from cells that line the milk ducts of the breast and then spread beyond the ducts. Inflammatory breast cancer progresses rapidly, often in a matter of weeks or months.*

Ok, besides this footnote on "Inflammatory Breast Cancer", the topics covered in this chapter are tied to the perils of chronic inflammation, cancer's sparkplug.

Phase 7
Dominance

At some point, like all living things, cancer wants to spread out and dominate its environment, like weeds in a maintained lawn.

Angiogenesis is the process by which a tumor attracts additional blood vessels to further nourish and accelerate its existence. Angiogenesis is an important natural process used for healing, and cancer cells use this to their advantage.

7a. Doctor Judah Folkman

In the 1970's, Doctor Judah Folkman of Harvard Medical became the father of angiogenesis research and treatment. Back in 1971, Doctor Folkman described tumors as "hot and bloody" and wondered how tumors were so adept in attracting such large flows of blood nutrients. What he discovered is that a certain enzyme triggers vascular growth.

Say you cut yourself and blood vessels are damaged. In the healing process this enzyme is produced locally to get vessels to grow into the new healing tissue. The formula for this enzyme is stored within the DNA of every cell, including cancer cells. The catch … Cancer cells release the angiogenesis enzyme unconditionally, and not just in the presence of damaged tissue.

For a tumor mass is to exceed 1 mm in diameter, additional vascularization must occur, and the secretion of angiogenic enzymes plays a major role in establishing a capillary & blood vessel network extended from the surrounding host tissue to the cancer tumor.

Since the 1970's, drugs to stem angiogenesis were developed as part of the standard treatment for certain tumor-based cancers.

7b. Angiogenesis Drugs

Today, there are over 20 such drugs that specialize in various cancer cell types, yet each drug inhibits only one aspect of the formation of new blood vessels, giving the tumors wiggle room to by-pass the drug. Plus, the drugs have toxic side effects.

Conversely, certain natural foods, though less potent, seem to stifle the various enzyme delivery paths cancer uses to attract new vessels.

And so, rather than taking problematic drugs, the idea of ingesting two or three natural angiogenesis inhibitors has merit, with the goal of thwarting the vascular development from *many* vantage points.

Because angiogenesis inhibitors work by slowing or stopping tumor growth without directly killing cancer cells, they are ingested over a long period, as other factors already described impinge the tumor. These natural products are low dose, but generally blanket the tumor, so long-term use puts up a meaningful obstacle for tumors attempting to extend their ranges.

There are multiple researchers digging into anti-angiogenesis. For example:

***The Angiogenesis Foundation in Cambridge Mass* is one.**

A detailed report from doctors S.M. Sagar, MD, D. Yance, MH, and R.K. Wong, MD, found in Current Oncology is also valuable in listing the natural substances that impede vascular growth, as follows.

- Curcumin
- Chinese Skullcap
- Resveratrol
- Grape Seed Extract
- Chinese Magnolia
- Milk Thistle
- Ginkgo biloba
- Quercetin

These can be purchased on-line and at health food stores. Remember, if a tumor cannot attract blood vessels, it cannot become dominant.

Phase 8
Metastasis

With metastasis, cancer spreads to other parts of the body and changes itself into different cell types. 90% of cancer deaths involve runaway metastasis, the cancer dominating the blood stream's nutrient supply. At some point, the body's trillions of cells experience dehydration and starvation. The same fate befalls the enfeebled immune cells. Often pneumonia sets in as the outcome.

So, you don't want this.

No one does, and so for both Conventional Medicine and Naturopathic Practitioners the purpose is to avoid reaching this point, or if at that point to arrest further advance. However, the two camps do not often cooperate with each other, so you need to be the one that works both sides of the isle.

Consider this: Before reaching the point of no return, over expanded cancer colonies depend completely upon the fixed, moment-by-moment nutritional resources the bloodstream offers and are therefore more easily deprived through dietary measures. And once diet deprives cancer cells and they become increasingly impotent, the billions of *empowered* immune system cells the body musters every second can help tip the scales, bringing death and destruction to the weakened colony day and night. More developed cancer may take longer to wear down, but it still remains vulnerable.

And do not forget the *infiltration* tactics where things cancer tumors hate can directly assail them without hurting the body – things such as heat, common baking soda, oxygen, green tea, saffron, CBD oil, and even frankincense. (And, chemotherapy)

Until now, your cancer resided on Easy Street, never facing all three frontal assaults. You never deprived it of sugar, even for a moment, your immune system never launched an all-out attack, and certainly natural poisons never infiltrated it making *it* feel sick every second of its existence.

Through *zero-sugar, empowered immune defenses,* and various *tumor infiltration tactics,* naturopathic countermeasures direct your body towards becoming a medical powerhouse able to impinge both current and future rogue cancer cells.

Once in a metastasis situation, though, the remaining option is chemotherapy, though it weakens the body further in order to blunt the cancer. If you go with chemotherapy (at any point in time), you need to do all you can on the naturopathic side of the equation to provide ballast for your little ship.

You can adopt naturopathic countermeasures before and after medical intervention to test and strengthen your body. Consider the following:

Often, with larger tumors in play, as a first step, Conventional Medicine may choose to shrink tumor(s) with a mixture of chemotherapy and radiation before surgery. This pre-surgery window can last three or four months, which is the perfect opportunity to introduce naturopathic countermeasures, doubling your weapons against the tumor (s).

If, say, your tumor is 2-3 cm, and the goal is to shrink it to 1 cm to allow for a lumpectomy rather than a mastectomy, but instead of 1 cm, the combination of Conventional and Naturopathic tactics brings you a .5 cm result, then a) you might postpone surgery for a few more months to see if further tumor reversal takes place, or b) you have the lumpectomy, knowing that naturopathic tactics are working, thereby providing some insurance against further outbreaks.

Don't give up on good health measures at any point just because you have outsourced some of your treatment to Conventional Medicine.

Remember, chemo is toxic, so even a two-to-three-week detox before getting the drug matters.

Supplement Appendix

As mentioned, there are a lot of supplements to take, but with multiple stages in cancer's trajectory, each stage requires both general use and specialized supplements, especially as we creep past age forty. After all, it is age that calls for supplementation to feed our tired and somewhat worn-out cells.

The alternative, accepting steady decline, should offset any complaints about the number of supplements, especially as supplements were mainly unknown throughout Western medicine until recent decades. We are lucky to have them.

But keep in mind, supplements are just one element of self-healing. Diet, energy boosting, detoxing, stress management, exercise, oxygen boosting and so on all come first. Don't get caught up with supplements thinking them a short cut that lets you off the hook.

A practical point follows ... once a week fill baggies or large pill boxes with a day's worth of AM and PM supplements. This way you will not be overwhelmed.

This appendix is organized using excerpts from the *Master Class Video Courses* which in more detail introduce the supplements as to what they are designed to achieve:

The protection of cells from viral attack (antiseptics & antioxidants),

Control over runaway auto-immune responses (anti-inflammatories),

Feeding the immune cells (for greater vibrancy in attacking antigens of any kind),

Reversing years of dense breast tissue accumulation (breast vascular support),

Containing glucose overloads (diabetic offsets),

Stemming blood vessel growth around tumors (stemming angiogenesis),

Destabilization of tumors (infiltration tactics), and

Enhancing the circulatory system (respiratory support).

To get you oriented, any supplements which can be purchased on *LifeExtension.com* have the LE inventory numbers indicated. Other supplier sites are also listed below.

Antiseptics & Antioxidants

Antiseptics in the blood stream are the first line of defense to weaken viruses entering the body, keeping them from infecting cells. Antioxidants are the second line of defense, and act as chemical shields protecting cell walls from oxidation (burning) by incoming oxygen molecules.

Oxidized cell walls allow viral penetration into the cell – a foothold for cancer.

LE# 01813 – Zinc – A key antiseptic weakening all viruses, including the coronavirus family.

LE# 01740 – Sea Iodine – A key antiseptic specifically supporting both the thyroid gland and the breast tissue. Iodine weakens the *cytomegalovirus* found in 100% of breast cancer tumors.

LE# 01436 – Blueberry Extract with Pomegranate – These concentrates provide the antioxidant benefits of these fruits without the sugar.

LE# 01533 – Vitamin "C", 500 units, twice daily. Take these religiously!

Doctor Bard's PMCaox Antioxidant Supplement – at *BardCancerCenter.com –* Doctor Bard is a leading diagnostic specialist for breast and prostate cancers and has developed an antioxidant supplement that reduces inflammatory triggers within these vulnerable tissue.

Anti-inflammatories

Runaway inflammation and autoimmune responses - where your own cells are considered to be antigens (viruses, bacteria, funguses, parasites and carcinogens) - confuse the resolve of your immune system, allowing viruses time to proliferate, while also stimulating cancer cells to divide. Anti-inflammatories interrupt this runaway inflammation trajectory, allowing the body to re-focus itself into eliminating true antigens.

LE# 02310 – Black Cumin Seed Oil & Curcumin Elite Turmeric Extract

Copaiba Oil – at *PlantTherapy.com* – Copaiba is an oil extracted from a South American tree which holds an organic molecule called beta-caryophyllene, a molecule that interferes with chronic inflammation patterns.

Copaiba Capsules – by do Terra – comes in pill form. One can ingest these, and use the oil topically over the tumor site.

Immune Support

The six primary immune cells include Antibodies, B Cells, T Cells, Neutrophils, Macrophages and Natural Killer (NK) Cells. Each has a specific role, but they also work in concert via enzyme signally amongst each other. They require their own set of nutrients to do the job.

LE# 01903 – NK Cell Activator – to awaken Natural Killer cells.

BETA 1,3D (Beta Glucan Vitamins) – at *TransferPoint.com* - Beta-Glucans act as an *immune-modulation agent,* meaning, they heighten the activity of the immune system. Immune attack cells grow more aggressive, and communication among the specialized immune cells becomes more emphatic, not unlike a basketball team suddenly shifting into "domination mode".

LE# 01708 – Reishi Mushroom Extract – The world offers many varieties of mushrooms, and many offer valuable nutrients not readily found elsewhere. But the red Reishi mushroom sits atop the heap with its various "active agent" molecules.

LE# 01751 – Vitamin D3 - Vitamin "D" focuses every cell in the body to fulfil its core mission – heart cells act as heart cells; bone cells act as bone cells, etc. The same is particularly true of the immune cells. Vitamin "D" keeps them focused.

Diabetes

Diabetic conditions – where sugar circulates for extended periods in the blood stream, enabling cancer - provides longer periods of sugar availability for the tumors. Sugar also causes glycation – the coating of blood vessels with a hard sugar residue. Both diabetes and glycation need to be arrested.

LE# 01625 – AppleWise – Offers the polyphenois found in apples without the sugar. Polyphenois offset sugar glycation of the blood vessels and temper inflammation.

Glucose Reduce – at *MedixSelect.com* – Glucose Reduce is a specially formulated natural dietary supplement, formulated by Dr. David Brownstein, containing 26 hand-picked ingredients. All these proven ingredients have been individually selected to help maintain optimal blood sugar, insulin, and cholesterol levels.

Taken before meals, Glucose Reduce a) triggers insulin production in the pancreas, and b) opens insulin/glucose receptors sitting on soft tissue cell walls – thereby accelerating absorption of sugars from the bloodstream, shortening sugar spikes.

Respiratory

Chronic inflammation, colds, the flu and corona viruses are respiratory conditions impinging lung function. As the lung loses efficiency, the heart is put under increasing pressure to compensate. The overall respiratory system can be provisioned as follows.

> *LE# 01733 – CoQu10/PQQ* – These co-enzymes are metabolized by the mitochondria in every cell. Mitochondria make energy for the cells, spinning at 2,000 revolutions per minute to do this, and they need the co-enzymes to keep up. Due to the heart's workload, heart cells have the most mitochondria in the body, so a heart under stress, more than all other cells, needs a robust supply of the two coenzymes.

> *LE# 02107 – Magnesium* – Magnesium is used in over 600 bodily functions, but in one key function it helps to keep blood vessels supple, allowing them to expand and contract in concert with the beating heart. Supple vessels take pressure off of the heart and deliver maximum oxygen to the body. Cancer hates oxygen.

> *LE # 02230 – Resveratrol* – Resveratrol is an organic molecule found in red grape skins, and it offers many advantages to the body, including keeping the circulatory system relaxed. This molecule sits behind what is referred to as the "French red wine effect", causing fewer heart disease issues in France than elsewhere. But it helps the immune response as well, also mitigating inflammation.

> *LE# 01982 – Super Omega 3* – This "fatty acid' controls excess triglyceride levels in the blood by parking triglycerides inside the fat cells until an "energy need" calls them out. Keeping them properly warehoused mitigates triglyceride overload in the bloodstream, one cause of heart disease. Omega 3 can be ingested through

fish, nuts and seeds, but a boost is probably needed by most people. Omega 3 is said to help with arthritic and depression issues as well. Also, pregnant woman need it to foster neurological development in the fetus.

Tumor Infiltration

Besides ingesting the honey/baking soda mixture described earlier in the book – which forces alkalinity consumption within the acidic tumors - other supplements can be taken that also disrupt cancer's comfort zone.

CBD Oil with Frankincense – at *BluebirdBotanicals.com* - CBD provides inflammation relief without the blood-thinning or stomach ulceration side effects that synthetic over-the-counter drugs cause. BLUE BIRD BOTANICALS sell a version infused with Frankincense, which disrupts cell division. You get two benefits in one by ingesting this oil under your tongue.

LE# 01432 – Optimized Saffron – Researchers have found that saffron, a spice of the Mediterranean diet, contains cancer-preventative properties, which include inhibiting tumor formation and preventing DNA switch mutations that activate cancer genes. Additionally, saffron has been shown to help reduce the harmful effects produced by chemotherapy drugs

Green Tea Blockers – at *Capsol-T.com* – Organic molecules in green tea plug cancer wall receptors listening for divide signals, thereby slowing or stopping the tumor's division rate. There are day time and "slow release" night time supplements available.

Nano Curcumin and Nano Quercetin – by One Planet Nutrition. By reducing inflammation, these supplements tamper down the angiogenesis buildup of blood vessels around tumors.

Dense Breast Cancer

After years of programmed cell division and cell death due to one's menstrual cycle, strands of scar tissue and collagen build up impinge blood flow support within the breast tissue. Density enables viral colonies to survive, increasing the possibility of cells being switched cancerous during the cell division copy step. But this accumulated fibrous tissue can be treated.

Doctor Bard's Primrose Oil – at *BardCancerCenter.com* – offers AM and PM mixtures.

Serraflazyme by *Cardiovascular Research LTD* – offers an enzyme that erodes dead scar tissue throughout the body, including breast tissue.

Myo-inositol – by – Zazzee Naturals – Acts as a restorative vitamin/enzyme for those living breast cells impinged by dense breast tissue. Doctor Blaylock recommends 500 mg capsules three times a day.

Betaine Anhydrous – by Nutricost – Reinforces the resolve of breast cell DNA, not to mutate cancerous during cell division. Doctor Blaylock recommends 750mg capsules twice a day.

Nano-Boswellia – by One Planet Nutrition – Reduces scar tissue and stems inflammation as it also triggers cell death within the tumor. Doctor Blaylock recommends 250 mg capsules three times daily.

LE# 02414 – Fisetin – Fisetin is an organic molecule found in apples, strawberries and other fruits that a) reverses cancer's avoidance of cell death, and b) works against cancer's ability to generate the angiogenesis enzymes which spur vascular growth around the tumor. In its natural form – eating apples and strawberries – the compound's presence is slight, but this supplement increases bio-availability by 25X, and delivers the compound without ingesting fruit sugars.

Other Suppliers

The following suppliers are recommended to complement the supplement program with physical, macro-boosting measures.

Saltworks – at Saltworks.com – offer a variety of bath salts delivered to your door.

VieLight – at VeiLight.com – offers an infrared light system that un-clumps our red blood cells which tend to bunch up with age, getting lazy. Autonomous red cells are re-awakened by VeiLight, bringing greater nutrient and oxygen provisions to functional cells operating at the capillary level.

Double Helix Water at *DoubleHelixWater.com* – Double Helix Water is a water with highly concentrated H^2O molecules. These molecules increase the electrical charge within your cells, adding vibrancy to cell defenses and cell healing.

NUTRITIONAL TESTING – Every bodily system processes, absorbs and metabolizes food (vitamins, minerals and nutrients) differently. Not everything ingested reaches the cells. NUTRITIONAL TESTING measures levels actually standing within the cells, not just the bloodstream, indicating where special supplementation is needed. For example, if your B12 level sits in the bottom 10% of the population, you need B12 supplements. There are at least 40 categories one can test for.

To address deficiencies (and allergies), find a naturopath to work with. They will organize various blood and urine tests to sort out your specific needs. Life Extension, Lab Corp and Quest all offer testing, but a naturopath should guide you.

LE# 02314 Two-Per-Day – Life Extension's "Two-Per-Day" multi-vitamin is indeed taken twice daily, and it covers many of the supplements mentioned in this chapter. One can rely solely on the multi-vitamin approach for day-to-day living and use precision supplements to boost any given vitamin or mineral should one's absorption level stay low (see testing above) or when fighting off a viral attack.

APPLE CIDER VINEGAR – by GOLI – Apple Cider Vinegar helps to lower glucose levels circulating in the blood stream, an natural offset to diabetes and cancer tumors. This gummy form can be used as a snack.

ACTALIN – Multivitamin by Medix Select - ACTALIN is a multivitamin specializing in thyroid health. Developed by Doctor Brownstein – a renowned specialist in thyroid and iodine issues – this pill contains 17 elements, including iodine. One should consider ACTALIN as part of a prevention plan.

Water – As most of your body is made up of water, one needs to obtain a source of clean water absent of contaminants or fluoride (a carcinogen that kills oral bacteria but affects every cell in the body). Tainted water of any kind inhibits the immune response against both invading antigens and internal cancer outbreaks. Water filters or purchased water solutions need to be implemented ASAP.

XYLTOL (natural sweetener) – A safe alternative to cane sugar, xyltol too comes from plants, but it has a different molecular configuration that cannot be converted into glucose by your digestive track. Because xyltol cannot morph into glucose, it not only by-passes anerobic-energy cancer cells, but it by-passes the entire glucose chemistry system, including the requirement of needing insulin to attach itself to normal aerobic-energy cells.

Epilogue

We hope that this ROADMAP provides you with a baseline perspective on the various countermeasures surrounding breast cancer.

Complementing the ROADMAP is the 320-page *Defeating Breast Cancer* book, which is a narrative of our journey in 2014, yielding more detail and a wider framework on the research.

Once you want to act, we recommend that you enroll in the 35-course *Master Class* video program, which further illustrates and fortifies the concepts covered herein, elevating them up to an actionable level.

After this, should you want support, instructors can be organized to move you forward. Support options are described on the *ManagingBreastCancer.com* web site.

Whether seeking prevention or treatment ideas, we wish the best for you, and hope that you can move forward with diminished fear.

Laura & Joe